Reflexology

*by A Guide To Hand & Foot Reflexology
- Diminish Stress and Pain Related
Disorders, Detoxify and Cleanse the
Body, and Improve Your Overall Health*

Table of Contents

Introduction

In literary terms, reflexology refers to the study of reflexes of human body. Reflexology is based on the ancient principle that each body part is directly associated to various reflex points in hands and feet via the neural network. Reflexology therapy techniques are derived from the fact that hands and feet can be used as shortcut maps for the entire human body.

This therapy practice suggests that each point on one's foot directly corresponds with a human organ and can be used to heal the problems associated with that specific organ. By pressing a relevant point on the foot or the hand, one can directly communicate with other body organs and heal them through massage therapies.

According to healing techniques documented by the ancient Chinese and Egyptians practitioners, each human body part can be represented by various reflex points located on hands and feet. By pressing these reflex zones, any issue related to the corresponding organ can be healed without the use of medication. Applying calculated pressure to these reflex zones create therapeutic effects in other parts of the body. The application of pressure on these zones stimulates the flow of positive energy through the nerves and helps in reducing pain.

Reflexology theories state that positive energy flows through a normal healthy body and helps in creating an upbeat nervous system. The flow of negative energy through the body affects the functioning of various organs. If negative energy is trapped in a certain body part, it results in accumulated stress in that specific organ. This stress is reflected as severe pain in that organ. The nerve endings from that region send the negative energy signals to the brain for interpretation which translates them as a call for help. Reflexology techniques help in releasing negative energy from the body to create a healthy internal environment.

An experienced reflexology specialist can diagnose an illness by handling the hands and feet of the patients. When a certain organ is ailing, the pain is reflected as a tender spot in the corresponding zone in the hands or feet. By examining these reflex zones, the reflexologist can determine the point from which pain is originating. Reflexology helps in getting rid of painful ailments through hand and feet massage therapies. Proper application of pressure in corresponding hand and feet zones helps in balancing the functioning of various organs and alleviates pain.

Application of gentle pressure in a firm manner on hand and feet zones stimulates the body organs and releases the effects of stress from them. Regular practice of reflexology techniques helps in maintaining a healthy mind which can regulate the nervous and circulation system for a healthy body.

The History of Reflexology

Modern reflexology is based on techniques used by people in ancient Egypt and China. Evidence supports that hand and foot therapy was being practiced in China in 4000 BC. The artwork found in tombs suggests that the same techniques were used in Egypt around the same time. Ancient art and inscriptions found in the tomb of Saqqara in Egypt depicts the discussion of a patient with the physician which translates as 'Don't hurt me', to which the practitioner's response is: 'I shall act so you praise me'. However the extent of similarity between ancient techniques and modern reflexology is not known.

The exact time and place of origin of reflexology cannot be articulated but the old art depictions date it back to a very long time ago. Reflexology has been in practice for a very long time in form of various therapies. Although modern reflexology might not be the direct ascendant of old techniques but it does derive its signature healing powers from them. The reflexes on our hands and feet play an important part in portraying the instinctive response of our body to an external stimulus. The identification of response points led to the start of hand and foot therapy for relieving pain.

Evidence suggests that the Chinese had divided the human body into longitudinal meridians to identify the stress points and to heal them. This division and detailed study led to the practice of body therapy. Modern reflexology dates back to the early 16th century when zone therapy techniques were published by various famous practitioners, including the work of Dr. Adamus, Dr. A'tatis and Dr. Ball. These early publications resulted in spreading the knowledge of zone therapy for treatment purposes.

The rediscovery of foot therapy is accredited to Dr. William Fitzgerald who used it to draw the attention of the medical world in early 20th century. He wrote various articles about the use of zone therapy for effective treatments for pain relief. Dr. Edwin Bowers encouraged him to publish his articles as a book. Dr. Fitzgerald published his first book 'Zone Therapy or Relieving Pain in the Home'. Dr. Fitzgerald later enlarged his book and published his work under the title 'Zone Therapy or Curing Pain and Disease '. He discovered that application of stress on various zones was not only an effective pain relief method but was also effective in pointing out the underlying causes.

Dr. Joe Riley was an admirer of Dr. Fitzgerald work and believed that reflex therapy has an immense impact on the human body. Miss Eunice Ingham, a physiotherapist working closely with Dr. Riley studied the work of Dr. Fitzgerald and performed her own experiments to validate and extend the findings. In the early 1930's, she took the opportunity to treat hundreds of patients using foot therapy and published her findings as a book entitled 'Stories the Feet Can Tell'. The collaboration of Eunice Ingham and Dr. Riley was responsible for bringing Dr. Fitzgerald's ideas to the outside world.

Eunice arranged workshops and seminars to shed light on the effects of foot therapy. She traveled around the world with his nephew Dwight Byers and laid the foundation of reflexology as we know it. Together they erected the National Institute of Reflexology where they further refined the techniques to offer effective relief from pain. Due to these improvements and publications, reflexology now stands as an important scientific technique that is today successfully implemented for effected therapy.

What Are the Benefits of Reflexology

Reflexology is helpful to people of all age groups. It is known to be an effective cure for a wide range of acute and chronic diseases including hormonal imbalance, back pain, spinal spasms, stress, migraines and circulatory problems. Based on the research studies conducted by various reflexology enthusiasts, some benefits of reflexology are penned below.

Stress Relief

Abrupt change in lifestyle, emotional situation and physical factors can cause hectic stress which can affect the mind and result in headaches, fatigue, and digestive problems. Hand and foot therapies of reflexology have a positive effect on brain activity and fight away these issues. It helps in avoiding depression and other side effects of prolonged stress.

Muscle Relaxation

Physical problems, too much heavy lifting and bad posture can cause muscles to spasm which can be highly painful. Reflexology techniques soothe the nerve endings to help the muscles relax. A few reflexology sessions can effectively calm exhausted muscles.

Pain Reduction

If right amount of pressure is applied on specific points on hands and feet, it effectively increases the flow of blood to the relevant nerve endings, soothing the sore muscles and curing body ache. Reflexology is a very effective pain management technique from which a huge number of patients benefit every day to get rid of long term ailments.

Circulation Improvement

A healthy body needs an efficient circulation of blood through the vessels. Lack of proper blood flow can affect in impaired body functions. Reflexology helps in soothing the tissues and blood vessels to allow uniform flow of blood to all parts of the body which strengthens the organs and rejuvenates fatigued tissues. Therapy techniques help in calibrating the communication between the nerves and blood vessels which helps in regulating the blood circulation. It helps in avoiding blood pressure problems in the elderly.

Chronic Sinus Infection

Controlled researches have suggested that reflexology helps alleviate pain in sinus infection and has same results as that of a nasal irrigation procedure. It helps in healing the swollen sinuses without the use of medication. Gentle application of massage on sinus zones on both hands and feet effectively reduces the pain caused by cold and flu.

Diabetes

Research studies conducted over controlled groups have revealed that reflexology has a positive effect on Type II Diabetes patients. It helps in regulating the blood circulation hence controlling the metabolism rate for the patient. Regular reflexology sessions can help regulate the production of insulin in the blood and affects the performance of pancreas. Reflexology can be very effective in lowering the pains of a long term diabetic patient.

Kidney Function

Foot reflexology regulates the renal blood flow which helps in removing the waste from blood to keep the body healthy. Regular foot reflexology increases the flow of blood to kidneys to keep the tissues fresh and active. Application of pressure on the renal zones helps in keeping up the performance of the kidneys. This is a very important and effective technique employed for patients with impaired kidney function.

Premenstrual Syndrome (PMS)

Premenstrual symptoms can be very stressful for women. Reflexology reduces the PMS effects and helps in lessening depression, anxiety and fatigue in women. Controlled group researches show that regular therapies help women in handling the PMS better. Use of foot zone therapy helps alleviating the pain in menstrual days and effectively reduced stress induced in the mind due to PMS pain.

Hormone Imbalance

Application of optimum pressure on the effective zones helps in regulating the hormone production in the body, thus maintaining a healthy amount of the required hormone level. Lesser production of required hormones by various glands affects the performance of various organs and can put a lot of stress on the mind. Reflexology helps in avoiding stress and side effects caused by hormonal imbalance. Release of endorphins and other hormones induced by therapy helps in calming down the nerve cells and improves their functioning.

Detoxification and Cleansing

Excessive bodily toxins can be harmful for health. Reflexology helps in clearing out the toxins that stagnate the body over time. Hand and foot therapy helps in eliminating the waste content to cleanse the body.

Apart from the ailments listed above, reflexology also has a positive effect on various other bodily problems. Proper use of reflexology therapies is known to have effectively cured depression, fatigue, pre / post cancer and seasonal allergies. Regular therapy sessions are important for getting rid of any issue. One simple massage is not effective in rooting out the problem entirely. Experiencing reflexology massages on a regular basis is bound to have a long lasting soothing effect on the body.

The application of soothing massage on hands and feet sends calming signals to the mind which helps in releasing stress and negative energy from the body. The extent of pressure applied depends on the level of pain that the body is enduring. The therapeutic effects of reflexology massages are countless and can be compounded if utilized frequently. Your body can benefit a lot from regular therapy sessions which help in rejuvenating dying cells and create a lively effect on you.

How Does Reflexology Work

Reflexology is a great help in soothing a variety of physical and muscular problems. It uses hand and foot therapy to release stress, regulate the blood circulation and to calm the nerves which in turn helps to get rid of pain. Various theories have been articulated to explain how reflexology works. Some common theories are penned down here.

The Nerve Impulse Theory

When a calculated pressure is applied to various zones of the foot or the hand, the afferent neurons conduct this impulse message to ganglia, the groups of neurons right outside our spinal cord. These nerve endings pass this message to the brain where it is interpreted and sends soothing sensations to the organs that are linked to the corresponding zones in the feet. It implies that reflexology works in vertical zones, that is if pressure is applied to a zone in the left foot, it will affect the corresponding organ only to which brain sends the interpreted signal. This theory is helpful in explaining how reflexology has a positive effect on those suffering from paralysis.

Gate Control Theory

The gate control theory explains pain as the subjective experience created by our brain in response to any external or internal stimulus. Apart from physical stimuli, the brain can also create a sensation of pain in response to emotional factors. A change in mood can be thus interpreted by the brain as a pain stimulator. Reflexology reduces stress, which results in an improved mood. A better mood helps in soothing the nerves which lessens the pain sensation. Hand and foot therapy controls the mind's perception of emotions to avoid pain.

Zone / Meridian Theory

Zone Theory is one of the most ancient theories used to explain reflexology. It states that the human body is divided into 10 vertical zones, and each zone corresponds to a specific point on the feet and hands. Every body organ is accessible through these zones and pressure application on zone points helps in soothing their corresponding organs. Carefully calculated pressure needs to be applied on the zones to heal the aching body part. An experienced practitioner can effectively apply pressure to these points to speed up the healing process.

Endorphin Release Theory

Bad energy accumulated in the body due to stress causes pain. Reflexology helps in emanating the stress channeled in these zones which results in better functioning of the organ. The reflexologist helps the patient release this bad energy by rubbing the various zones in feet and hands. This process releases endorphins in the body which help in creating a soothing and calming effect on the mind and helps in numbing the pain. Endorphins are body's natural pain killers which help in soothing without any side effects. Reflexology helps in increasing the release of endorphins to alleviate pain.

Impeded and Unimpeded Energy Flow Theory

Above theory suggests that the ground is comprised of positive and negative energies which can be picked by human body while walking. The pulsating energies from the ground can be transferred to the human body via feet in the form of electrical charge. The energy receptors of the feet pick these signals and send them to the brain for interpretation. The blockage of energy passageways can sometimes results in energy congestion.

Negative energy thus acquired can get congested in the brain if not let out. Reflexology helps in unblocking the natural passageways so that negative energy can be emanated from the body to give it a calming effect. After foot therapy, negative energy is released back to the ground through the energy passageways of the feet. Regular therapy keeps negative energy from accumulating in the body so that the mind remains fresh and stress-free all the time, giving you a soothing sensation.

Above are some of the theories that are used to describe this particular massage therapy technique. Other common theories formulated by reflexology practitioners include the electric impulse theory, facilitation theory, feet U bend theory and many others. Science hasn't rooted out the main root behind this effective zone therapy but evidence suggests that all above theories collectively support the concept of reflexology.

Each of these theories implies that stress and negative energy can have a huge downing effect on the mind which is sometimes perceived as physical pain. It is important to get rid of negative energy to minimize the risk of various other diseases. Regular reflexology sessions can have a great impact on the brain and help in regulating the neurological and hormonal system of the human body. Consulting an established reflexology expert will help you locate the origin of negative energy in your body and will alleviate pain from various body parts.

The Structure of Feet

Foot Reflexology Chart Map (Diagram)

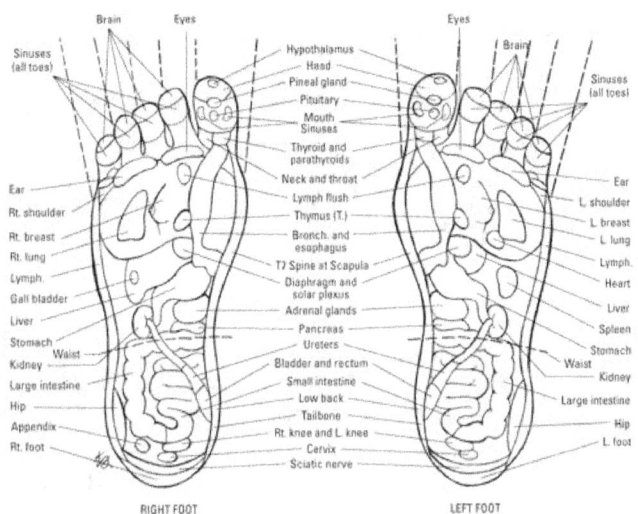

The above chart depicts the various reflex points of the foot. Stress, anxiety, sleep disorders and muscle spasms can be healed by rubbing or applying pressure to the zones corresponding to each organ. Careful application helps in calming down the nerves.

Problems relating to feet

Each toe and finger belongs to the corresponding body organ. If a body part is diseased, it imparts its effect on the corresponding zone on the feet. Sore feet can be used to diagnose various diseases that may have an effect on these zones.

To diagnose a disease, a foot therapist applies impulsive pressure with a rubber hammer or a blunt probe to pin point the origin of pain. The nerves communicating with the diseased body part show more sensitivity which results in a sudden surge of pain. This surge of pain in a specific zone of the foot helps in diagnosing the organ from where the pain is originating. Various problems have been attributed to be cured by foot therapy. Some main problems that can be handled using foot reflexology are:

Insomnia

Insomnia is directly related to increased stress level in the system. The nerve endings in the finger tips of the toes directly correspond with the section of the brain that deals with stress issues. By carefully applying pressure on the toe tips with the help of fingers help in regulating the mind and creates a tranquilizing effect. Regular foot therapy helps in completely ruling out insomnia even in long-term patients.

Abdominal pain

Digestive issues and intestinal disorders often result in severe abdominal pain. Medicines may have side effects but reflexology techniques help in eliminating the main cause of this pain. By employing therapy techniques on the large intestine's zone on the foot, the organ can be stimulated to perform its job properly so that you won't have to suffer from immense abdominal pain in the future.

Stomach Disorders

Stomach disorders are usually related to stress or changes in one's emotional state. A sudden revelation or a bad news can badly affect your nervous and digestive system which results in reduced appetite. By applying reflexology techniques on the stomach zone of both the feet, you can get rid of this problem. It helps in restoring yoru digestive system back to its original performance so that you can enjoy healthy meals.

Sinus Infection

The lower parts of toes correspond directly with the nerve endings in the sinuses. Increased production of sinus fluid by the glands results in flu and cough. A reflexologist can help you get rid of your sinus problem by rubbing these zones on your feet so that sinus glands can operate on an optimum level. It helps in relieving the body from pain caused by excessive production of fluid.

Liver problems

Sudden surges of pain in the lower abdomen can be attributed to liver disorders. Since liver is a very important body organ, it is important to take notice of such pain immediately. If medicine doesn't seem to be effective, you can contact a reflexologist for foot therapy which results in effective healing of liver issues.

Foot Care

As the above section explains, a number of diseases and issues can be cured by simple foot therapy. In turn, applying stress on a certain zone on the feet can also cause pain in the corresponding organ. People tend to take care of their hands and face but usually forget to nurture their feet. Foot care plays an important role in your health. Healthy feet are an important attribute of a healthy body.

To avoid diseases caused by feet, proper care is required. Being over-weight is an important factor that affects your feet badly. Putting too much weight on yoru feet affects their withstanding ability and lowers down their stamina. This can cause regular pain in the feet. Pain induced in different zones can affect the corresponding body organ. Thus one tiny issue leads to a whole new chapter of diseases. By avoiding these small problems, you can ensure that your feet are in best shape, which helps in taking your first steps towards your health.

Feet require proper cleaning to stay healthy. Often people neglect their feet when taking a shower which is definitely not the right approach. For healthy feet, scrub your feet during each shower you take to ensure all dirt particles and bacteria are effectively removed. Properly cleaned feet will help you establish a healthy body structure.

Structures of Hand and Wrist

Hand Reflexology Chart Map (Diagram)

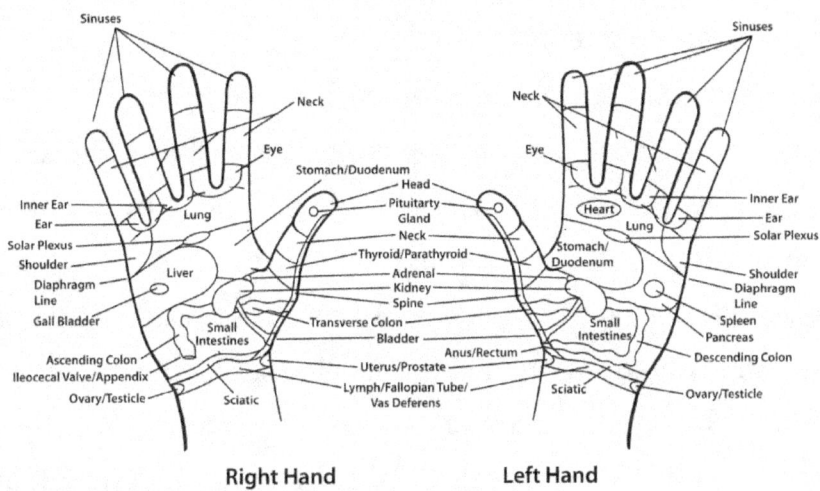

Right Hand   Left Hand

The zones indicated on both hands correspond to the respective organ. Each point on the left hand directly corresponds to the organs located on the right side of the body. The right hand is responsible for communicating sensations to the organs on the left side. Stress and circulation problems can be handled by applying pressure to corresponding zones.

The benefit of understanding hand reflexology techniques is that you can try this yourself as well since it is easy to access and massage hands. By looking at a hand reflexology chart, you can locate the reflex points for different organs. Many reflex points on the palms mirror the reflex points on the top of your hands. By accessing these points, you can massage the tense nerves to heal yourself.

Problems relating to the hand

The organs directly related to the corresponding zones on your hands can be healed by massaging the respective zones. Each organ represented by your hands can be healed by accessing your hands. The thumbs represent your head and can be used to get rid of a severe headache. By accessing your finger tips, you can lessen down your sinus problems. Similarly the inner palms relate to stomach and lung problems. Some main problems which can be healed using hand reflexology methods are mentioned below.

Digestion Issues

Stress and poor blood circulation can often result in a weak digestive system. Hand reflexology can be used to effectively regulate oxygenated blood and to support the digestive system. By massaging the hands, you can stimulate the intestines for better absorption of food. To solve digestive issues, it is advised to interlock the ringers of both hands and to roll the reflexology probe round in the lower palms. Regular practice of this reflexology exercise helps in getting the digestive system back on track.

Cold and Flu

Cold and flu basically affect you due to poor defense mechanism of your head and sinuses. Therefore for healing flu, you need to focus on the head and sinus reflexes of your body. Locate the sinus points of your fingers to cure a severe cold. Massage your fingers from the base to the tip of each several times. By performing this technique on both hands several times a day, you'll soon get rid of flu. Regular application of pressure on these points will help you avoid catching flu later even in a severe cold weather.

Insomnia

Accumulation of disturbing thoughts in the mind leads to an upsetting mental state. An upset mind finds it hard to sleep effortlessly at night. Irregular performance of any of the body parts can also result in insomnia. It can usually be cured by stimulating the activity of the pituitary gland. You can rub the middle of your thumbs to decrease your insomnia.

Apply pressure on the middle of your thumb using the nail of the other thumb. Constant pressure application for about 45 seconds to one minute is bound to relax your entire body to help you with insomnia. By performing this easy exercise on both thumbs several times a day you can entirely get rid of insomnia issues. Make it a regular practice to avoid insomnia in the future.

Back Pain

Back pain is usually caused by poor regulation of the spine. To stimulate your spine, you need to massage the outer sides of your palms. The thumbs side of your hand down to the wrist is directly in correspondence with the spine. To stimulate a reflex response from the spine, you need to massage these areas of your hand. A reflexologist can handle this situation by starting from the top of the thumb all the way down to the wrists. By gently rubbing this area, the spine can be aroused to move back in place. Regular reflexology hand massages can help reduce back pain in the long term.

This exercise needs to be repeated several times a day to avoid severe back pain. You can also learn this technique from your reflexologist to help heal yourself. Back pain can cause tender spots on the sides of your wrists. When applying pressure to these spots, you may need to be careful. If rubbing these parts is painful, don't apply too much pressure. Controlled pressure will help you heal faster.

Low Libido Problems

Hand reflexology can help stimulate the fertility organs. If you are having pain in ovary or testes area, you can use hand therapy to cure it. The lower libido healing technique can be used the patient himself/herself easily. To heal such a problem, hold your wrist with a thumb and finger, forming a ring around it. Grasp the wrist in such manner firmly and twist it softly. Applying too much pressure when twisting might harm your wrist. Grab the wrist softly and twist it 15-20 times using your other hand. Continuous twisting will help stimulate the ovary / testes and prostate and heal your problem.

The practice needs to be performed on both the hands to achieve effective results. You can repeat this process twice a day to alleviate the pain. Regular use of this reflexology technique will ultimately end your problems.

Hand Care

Healthy hands are beacons of a healthy body. Tense hands can send upsetting signals to various organs of the body that correspond to the zones in your palm. It is important to keep your hands in good shape so that they won't induce any negative energy on any other body part. A simple reflexology massage can help in releasing tension from hands for a balanced system. It is important to induce relaxation in your palms so that organs associated with palmer zones can be relieved from any accumulated negative energy.

For a relaxed mind, you can use reflexology techniques to calm down the nerves. Start with yoru finger tips and pinch each one by applying slight pressure using your thumb and index finger. Application of pressure for a few seconds on each finger will help create a soothing sensation in the nerves. Next you need to squeeze the sides of yoru fingers in a similar fashion. It helps in unblocking the paths for negative energy to let it flow out of your body. You can rub the fingers vigorously from their roots back to the tips. Continue this massage for a few minutes for a promising result.

After rubbing the fingers, you need to massage your palms. Put your palms together and squeeze them together. Rub them against each other to regulate the blood flow in the body. For better results, use your thumbs to gently rub the inner palms.

You can start from the inner side of your palms and spread the massage outwards. Gently rubbing the palms has a very calming effect on the nerve endings in this area. Use opposite thumbs to massage both the hands in this manner. Taking deep breaths while massaging the hands will help in relaxing the mind and the body.

Trying this hand massage technique on a regular basis will help you release stress and keep it from accumulating in your mind. A relaxed mind will be more efficient in taking care of the body and will help in reducing the risks of catching various stress related issues. Hand reflexology helps in improving the functioning of various body parts and assists in alleviating the pain caused by current ailments. Hand reflexology can also help in putting an end to long term ailments.

Pressure Points

Besides the feet and hands, the other important part for reflexology treatments is the ear. A large number of reflexology pressure points have been described in the ear. Just as in the case of the feet and hands, applying pressure to these ear reflex areas can relieve symptoms like migraine headaches, attention deficiencies as well as contributing to pain relief, clearing infections, lowering blood pressure and balancing hormones. The ear provides suitable reflexology zones due to it is extensively enervated structure. It is believed that more that 100 specific reflex points can be found in the ear, with these points bearing close linkages with the internal organs of the body on one hand and the musculoskeletal system on the other. The pressure points of the ear relate to energy centers known as meridian.

Basically, the ear is composed of three parts: the external ear, the mid ear, and the internal ear. Although each ear is unique and bear a specific signature per individual, there are cross-cutting characteristics that can be located in every ear, and that also help in identification of reflexology pressure points and standardization of reflexology protocols. Each ear has four prominences, three depressions, four notches, and one ear lobe on the anterior surface of the auricle. The posterior surface of the auricle on the other hand is characterized by three flat areas, five grooves, and four prominences.

Two different reflexology maps have been developed for the ear's pressure points, one showing the pressure points connected to the body's internal organs, and the other for points used for external body parts targeted therapy.

The ear is exceptional in that each ear has a complete reflex map of the body, transversed with a rich nerve network and multiple connectors to the central nervous system. Another unique feature that distinguishes ear reflexology zones from those of the feet and hands is the projection of the inverted fetal position on the outline of the ear's pressure points.

The regions of both the head and the neck are located in the ear lobe while the legs are located at the opposite end. The soft location where most people have their cosmetic ears piercing is the point for the eye reflex.

Pressure points along the outer part of the ears are associated with both the lower and the upper extremities. At the folds of the outer part of the ears are the pressure points that are lined to the pelvis, back, hips, and even the neck. At the regions around the middle of the ears but not down in the ear canal, and the region where the jawline meets the ears have a connection with specific organs and parts of the body that control our hunger. The point in the ear, famously referred to as point zero, has been shown by numerous reflexology therapists to play a role in restoration of homeostatic balance in the body. The point zero not only balances energy of the body, but is also used to regulate the brain, viscera, and hormones.

It is generally agreed that the auricular therapy and reflexology mappings often overlap. These points are in the order of hundreds, however, some of the vital points besides point zero that have received increased interest in reflexology therapy include:

- The Shen Men, also referred to as 'Divine Gate', is considered to be so powerful that it is used in treatment of almost all conditions from stress to anxiety, depression, inflammatory diseases and many others.
- The autonomic point which is used to balance the sympathetic and parasympathetic nervous systems as well as blood circulation.
- Thalamus point is targeted for over excitement, shock and sweating.
- Endocrine point is used to balance endocrine hormones, hypersensitivity and rheumatism

- Master oscillation point plays a role in balancing the left and right cerebral hemispheres, often for left-hand oriented individuals.
- Allergy point is targeted to reduce allergic inflammatory reactions and eliminate toxicity.
- Tranquilizer point is useful for general sedation and anxiety.
- Master sensorial or 'eye' point is helpful in addressing tinnitus and blurred vision
- Master cerebral point is critical for nervousness, anxiety and fear problems.

Besides the three main reflexology zones, that is feet, hands and the ear, there are other regions that also have important pressure points for reflexology therapy.

For instance, in treatments of knee pains commonly caused by osteoarthritis, bursitis, muscle strains, tendonitis, serious injuries to cartilage and ligaments, the knee reflex point which is located in a small soft triangular section located just below the bone of the ankle, is targeted to strengthen the knee joint and heal any injuries in this knee area. The calf's nose pressure point is placed just outside the knee cap and is targeted to relieve knee stiffness and pain. Reflexology on the nourishing valley pressure point, which can be felt as a hollow between the tendons at the edge of the knee crease, helps address knee pain, tummy ache as wells as genital disorders. Then there is the interesting 'three mile' pressure point located two inches below the kneecap and just one away from the shinbone which helps in strengthening the whole body besides relieving knee pain. The 'commanding activity' reflex point, located at the edge of the fold on a knee (bent), will aid in relieving almost all knee pains.

One pressure point known as 'shady side of the mountain', located on the inside of the leg, just below the bulge on the head of the shin bone, is considered a miracle. Through it, reflex can be achieved for several health conditions in the body like water retention problems, knees difficulties, swelling, leg tensions, varicose veins, cramps, edema and urinary tract abnormalities. Thumb and Index Finger joint (the joint between the thumb and index finger) is an important pressure point that can help relieve any kind of pain in the body as well as in reducing excess heat in the body.

Hand Reflexology - Techniques and Tips

Performing hand reflexology has one advantage owing to the easy accessibility of the hands; it is therefore easy to administer a self-massage on the hands following basic reflexology techniques. However, one fact to contend with is that reflexes lie much deeper under the skin, which means one must reach deeper and hold for longer to stimulate the hand reflexology points. It will therefore take a longer time to achieve the result by hand reflexology but the procedure remains as effective as the others.

The hand reflexology technique involves using one finger or the thumb to apply pressure on one spot of the hand and then rotating the finger on the same spot for about five seconds before lifting the finger and transferring to new adjacent spots till the whole finger is covered according to the hand reflexology protocol. It is advisable that the thumb / finger nails of the person carrying out the reflexology should not be too long as this will to exert painful pressures, nor cut too short as to be unable to cause any pressure at the desired points.

It is critical to note that the first important phase of hand reflexology is the relaxation phase. This phase helps to set the right tone for the treatment and helps to soothe the muscles before the therapeutic deeper massage of the reflexes begins. It is recommended that you work on the right hand to the end before moving to the left.

I.

The relaxation exercise can be done by simply following the procedures described below:

- Apply little oil or cream around the wrist to lubricate the hand and gently massage with slow outward-sweeping motion of your thumbs.
- Transition into the palm, keeping the same motion and massaging slowly for about 30 seconds from the center of the palm slowly to the edges.
- Turn over the hand so that the palm faces down and gently use the thumbs to massage across the top of the hand, starting from the areas between the knuckles to the wrist. Too much pressure may lead to pain hence the caution for gentility.
- Then hold the finger at the base and gently twist it side to side so as to slowly rotate the knuckle bone joint. Slide the massaging hand up the finger to the second joint and do the same process. Repeat this procedure as you move up to the top joint of the finger. Do this process for the other fingers also, one at a time.

- Finally, gently squeeze the right hand and pat off the oil with a towel.

The hand reflexology procedure can then proceed to the next steps.

II.

This step is aimed at stimulating the hand meridians:

- Using the hand reflexology technique described earlier, apply pressure for three to five seconds, in a clockwise and then anti-clockwise direction, on each meridian point located at the distal ends of the fingers.

III.

Working on the fingers:

- Working from the tip to the base, move line by line, from the inside to the outside, all around the entire thumb.
- From the thumb, move to the index finger and repeat the above tip to base motion, and then proceed to all other fingers on the right hand. Every part of the fingers should be well covered.

IV.

Palm of the hand:

The best hand position for this step is the right hand laying flat on a table or an alternative soft surface with the palm facing upwards. Then follow the steps listed below till the hand is completed.

- Begin the hand reflexology technique on the soft padding under the fingers. You should do this first downwards, then upwards, and lastly sideways. Move on to the center of the palm and repeat the same pattern.
- Then using the same technique and pattern as above, do the outer edge of the hand from base of the little finger to the wrist.
- Repeat the same technique and pattern to do reflexology from the base of the thumb across to the outer edge of the hand, line by line, till the entire soft padding between the palm and wrist is covered. This is a critical area as it is connected to many vital body parts including the spine and digestive system.
- And lastly, very gently and softly rub the wrist once from left to right, then once in the opposite direction.

IV.

Working on the back of hand:

For this step, it is preferable that the hand is turned over so that the palm faces down. The same hand reflexology technique is used here but with more gentle touch. Frequently confirm from the person receiving reflexology if they are comfortable with the amount of pressure being applied as this is a highly sensitive area and caution must always be taken to ensure gentle pressure is used.

- Using unidirectional motions, work downwards from the knuckles of the hand to the wrist. Repeat this until every part of the back of the hand has been done, then gently carry out reflexology technique around the wrist bone and along the wrist.

VI.

After completing the right hand, turn to the left hand and repeat step I up to step V on it.

VII.

Final relaxation of the hand:

- Just at the end of step V on the left hand, while it is still facing palm down, apply a small amount of massage oil or cream to the skin, and gently massage for about 30 seconds, moving in a knuckles to the wrist direction. Also rubdown around the wrists for 10 to 15 seconds.
- Turn the hand up side down and gently massage across the palms with your thumbs. You may apply some oil or cream if need be.
- Lastly wring out each finger gently and turning to the right hand, repeat the relaxation exercise.

VIII.

Drinking water:

Water is an important component of the reflexology procedure as an increase in the rate of excretion of wastes occurs. Plentiful amount of water is therefore recommended, a big glass immediately and much more during the rest of the day, to facilitate the washing away of any excess body wastes from the blood system. Accumulation of such wastes may lead to a 24 hours of flu like symptoms

Foot Reflexology - Techniques and Tips

Foot reflexology is method for achieving quicker results as the pressure points of the feet are very close to the skin.

The most common method for conducting foot reflexology techniques is referred to as thumb-walking. It is very important to learn how to do the thumb-walking and how to identify which part of the thumb to use. The method is common because it easy, you just flex the thumb towards the palms and straighten it, and by repeating the two actions over and over, the thumb simply 'walks' forward. The techniques are also very easy and effective. In addition, thumb-walking is also valued for allowing a reflexologist to apply stimulating pressure to every single part of the foot, potentially covering all the pressure points on the foot and thereby giving not only a very effective but also a relaxing reflexology treatment.

You can learn to determine which part of the thumb to use by simply:

- Holding both your hands together, palm to palm, with the fingers on the right hand corresponding to those on the left. Then focusing on the top part of the thumbs, slightly roll the thumbs till the two thumb nails get in touch with each other. You should be able to feel the inside edge of the very top of your thumbs where the two meet each other. That is the part used for thumb-walking.

The thumb-walking technique is a simple procedure. You can easily learn and perform it by following the steps summarized below:

- Simply get any object and place the thumb in a manner that the part of the thumb for doing thumb-walking, as described above, is in touch with the object.
- Flex your thumb and simply unbend it over the object without moving the object itself. By repeating the flexing and straightening actions with the thumb kept in contact with the object, you will notice that not only does your thumb creep forward slowly, but you are actually exerting some pressure on the object at the point where your thumb is held in contact with it.
- You can now try to apply more pressure when straightening the thumb for greater effect. You can practice this technique on both thumbs till it becomes easier and faster.

Once these techniques are learned, the actual feet reflexology process can easily be carried out. The right foot is the favorite foot to begin with.

I.

Relaxation of the feet:

- Take the first 30 seconds massaging the foot. Work on all the surface of the foot with slow but firm massaging, beginning at the toes and moving to the heels.

- Hold the foot at the spine with the thumbs on the lower side and the fingers on the upper surface and gently wring the hands, from the mid region, away from each other. This will slightly twist the foot at the spine region towards one direction, change the direction and repeat the exercise for 30 seconds to produce the adequate relaxation.

II.

Thumb-walking the spine:

- Use the thumb-walking techniques learned above to walk along the spine, first in the heel to toes direction and then in the reverse direction. Change the direction once again by walking the spine in short distances across from right to left on the inner side.

III.

Rotation of the toes:

The next step is to rotate the toes, beginning with the big toe and continuing, toe by toe, until the little end toe. This is carried out by:

- First holding the toe firmly at the base joint where the toe attaches to the foot, and then gently moving your hands in circular motions. By this, you will be rotating and stretching the toe at this base join.
- Move to the point just above the second joint of the toe and repeat the circular motion described above, and lastly rotate the very top joint in the same manner.

It is interesting to note that the human cranial bones are separate bones fused at the sutures, which are in communication with the toe joints, hence by rotating the toes in this exercise, extra blood circulation is directed to these skull bone joints.

IV.

The meridian points:

All the toes of the foot, apart from the middle toe, have meridian points located at the end of the toes, just around the root of the toe nails. The big toe has such points on either edges.

- Focusing on the location of these meridian points, hold the toe with one hand and apply pressure at the meridian points with one finger in a circular clockwise motion, then change to the reverse direction.
- Continue with the process for 10 seconds for each toe, starting from the big to the little toe.

V.

The next step is to thumb-walk the toes:

- As learnt before, do the thumb-walking techniques on the toes starting at the base and moving upwards in a straight line to the tip. Repeat the process till all sides of each toe is covered, always beginning from the big to the little toe.

Always inquire from the person receiving the reflexology exercise to know the extent of pressure that is bearable, incase the person is feeling too much pain, break for while.

VI.

This step focuses on the chest area:

- Gently thumb-walk the whole surface of the ball area of the foot, first in an upwards direction, then downwards and lastly in an angle.

VII.

The top and back areas of the foot:

- With the foot sole facing down, thumb-walk from one end (toes) to the other end (ankle) till the whole top surface of the foot is covered.

- Now change direction and thumb-walk across the entire top surface of the foot from right to left.

This part of the foot may be very sensitive in some people.

VII.

The liver / stomach area of the foot:

- Thumb-walk on an angle across the area between the chest of the foot and above the waistline. Turn to the opposite angle and repeat.

This area is connected to the liver and stomach, with respect to the foot you are handling.

IX.

The intestinal area of the foot:

- This area is located around the waistline and the pelvic area of the foot and it is connected to the large and small intestines. Thumb-walk across the foot at an angle on the intestinal region then turn to the opposite angle and repeat.

X.

The pelvic area of the foot:

- Thumb-walk in a left to right direction over the pelvic area ensuring you adequately cover both left and right sides of the heel, then do the same for the back of the heel.

- Finish with a gentle massage of the whole foot for about a minute to relax the foot.

XI.

The left foot:

- After completing the right foot, turn to the left foot and repeat step I to step X on the left foot.

XII.

Drinking water:

As in the hand reflexology, drinking plenty quantity of water after the foot reflexology therapy is extremely important as it facilitates the removal of wastes from the body. The person receiving reflexology treatment should therefore drink one big glass of water immediately after the exercise and drink much more in the following 24 hours.

Conclusion

Reflexology plays an important role in reducing stress and the implications caused due to immense stress. Reflexology practitioners believe that the patient also plays a vital role in recovery. Theories suggest that the job of the therapies is to facilitate the patient in releasing negative energy and stress effects from the body. A therapist helps in the patient in letting stress out and assists in inducing a tranquilizing effect in the brain for a serene mind. Hand and foot zone therapies are used to stimulate the nerves to create a calming sensation. Reflexology facilitates the repairing process for human body by controlling the emotional side of the brain.

Accumulation of unwanted energy in body parts leads to diseases. The use of therapy techniques helps in releasing this energy so that the body can nurture itself. A practitioner can actually feel the flow of energy in the body and use it to emanate the low feelings. If the practitioner employs the massage techniques in the right manner, even the patient can sense the movement of negative energy vibes in body trying to get out of the system. Proper massage helps in unblocking the passageways for this built up energy and releases it out to relax the mind and the body.

The lack of body's ability to produce the regulated amount of hormones also leads to a number of stress related problems.

Reflexology helps in regulating the hormonal flow to ease the healing process. By consulting an experienced reflexology practitioner, you can finally wave goodbye to these old hormone related problems to rid your body of minor issues that result in bigger health problems.

Therapeutic techniques take into account both the physical and emotional stress of the body to induce relaxing sensation. Relaxed nerves calm down the emotions and release the mind from irrelevant stress. A calm mind helps in soothing the organs and repairs the emotional and physical damage induced by stress and circulation problems. An experienced practitioner can help you enjoy the calming effects of reflexology to help you avoid neurological and physical issues caused by stress.